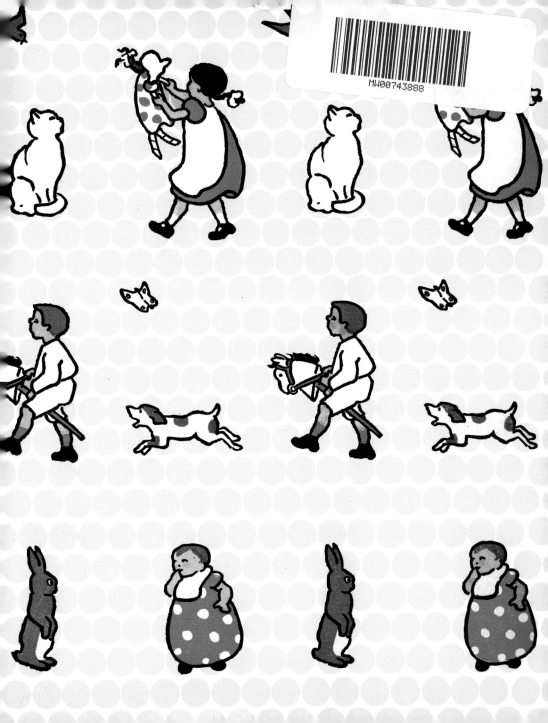

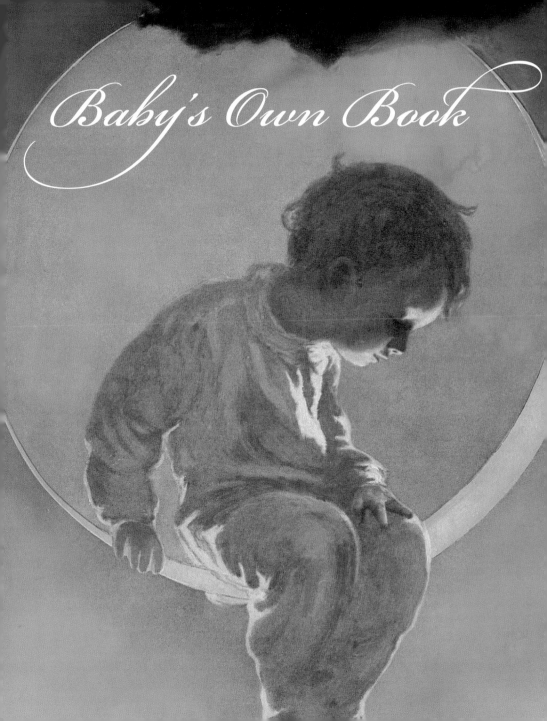

Baby's Own Book

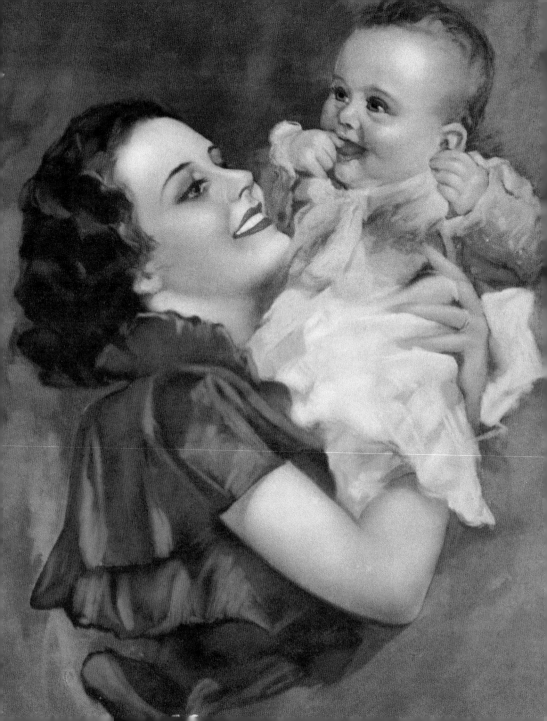

Baby's Own Book

BABY'S FIRST YEAR

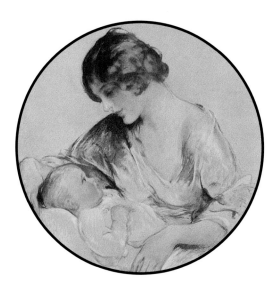

COMPILED BY BLUE LANTERN STUDIO

LAUGHING ELEPHANT

MMIV

COPYRIGHT © 2004, BLUE LANTERN STUDIO

ISBN 1-883211-36-0

PRINTED IN CHINA THROUGH COLORCRAFT LTD., HONG KONG

LAUGHING ELEPHANT BOOKS

3645 INTERLAKE AVENUE NORTH   SEATTLE, WASHINGTON   98103

WWW.LAUGHINGELEPHANT.COM

THE BABY BOOK OF:

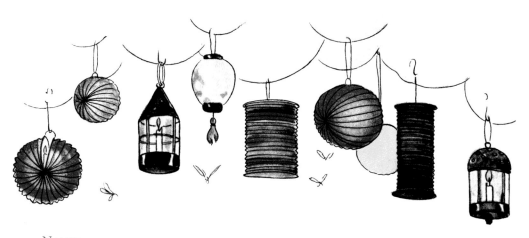

NAME:

BIRTH DATE: TIME:

PLACE:

CITY: STATE:

PARENTS:

ATTENDANTS:

MEASUREMENTS:

WEIGHT: HEIGHT:

VISITORS . . .

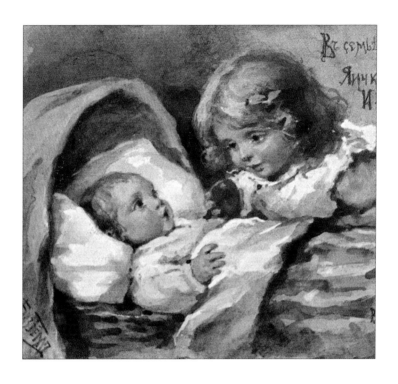

AND WHAT THEY SAID

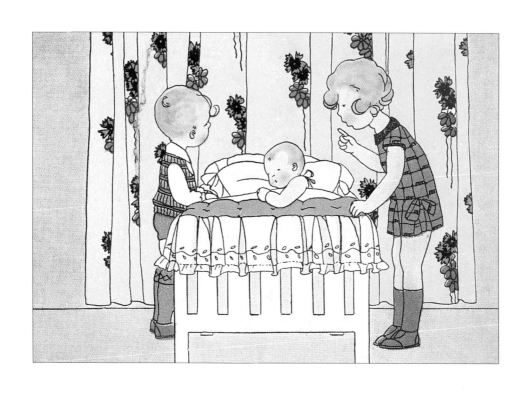

MEASUREMENTS & IMMUNIZATIONS

DATE: | HEIGHT: | WEIGHT: | IMMUNIZATIONS:

GIFTS

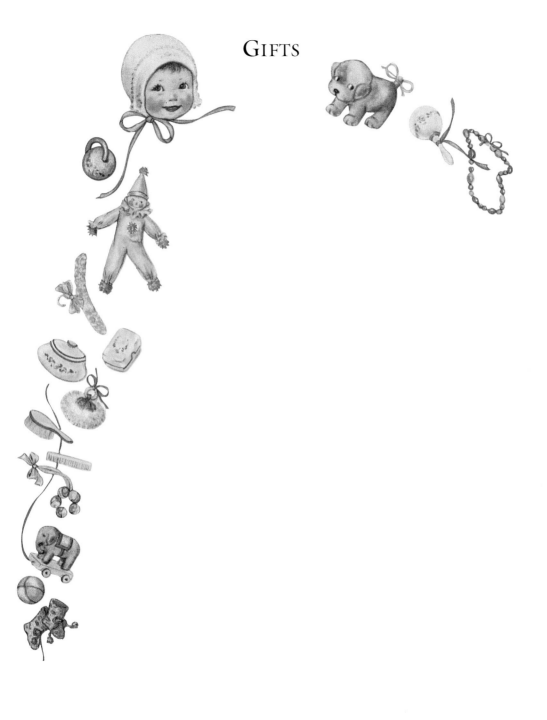

BABY SMILES

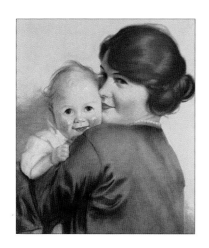

DATE:

Baby's Bath

Date:

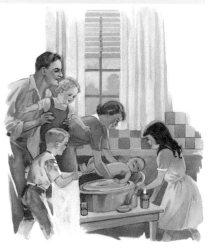

Baby's Friends

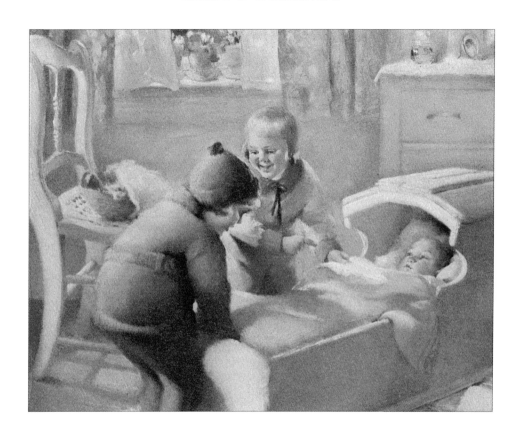

Baby's Friends

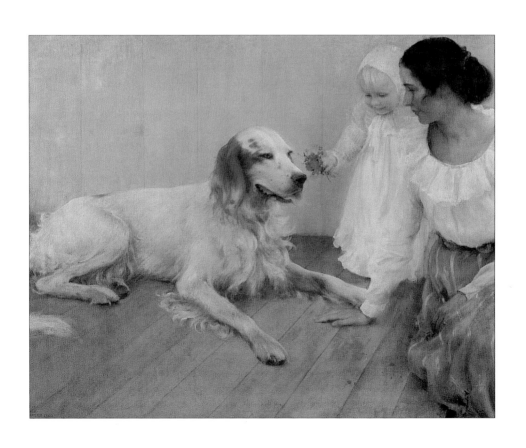

BABY SITS UP

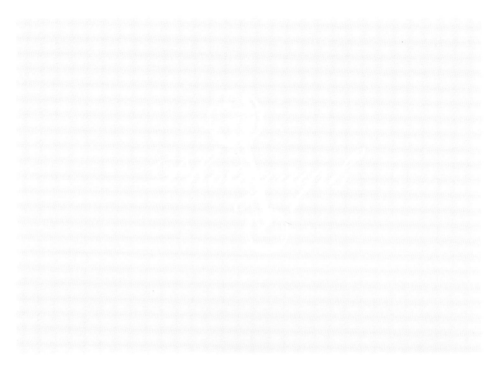

DATE:

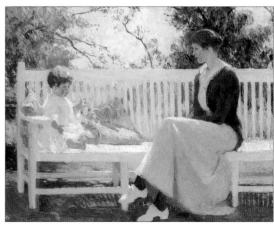

MILESTONES

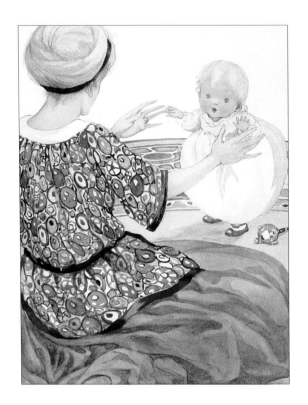

BABY CRAWLS • DATE:

BABY STANDS • DATE:

BABY WALKS • DATE:

Favorite Foods

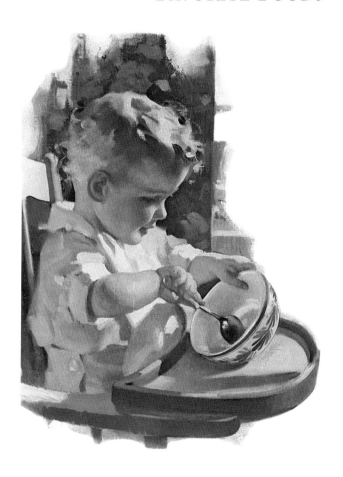

First Hair Cut

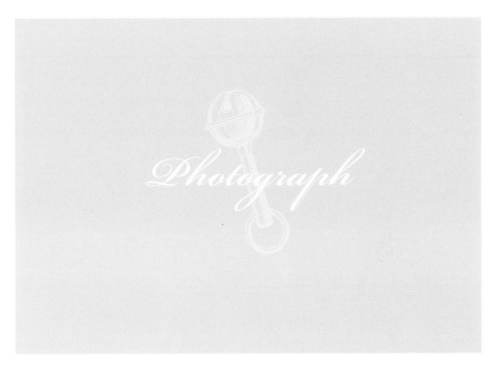

Date:

Lock of hair

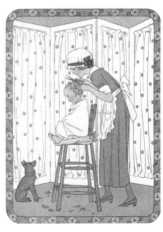

BABY SPEAKS

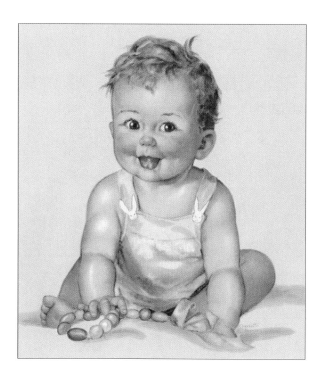

FIRST WORDS:

1.

2.

3.

4.

5.

6.

7.

8.

9.

10.

MEMORABLE SAYINGS:

First Outing

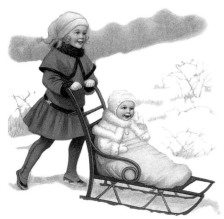

Date:

Where:

Baby's Games & Toys

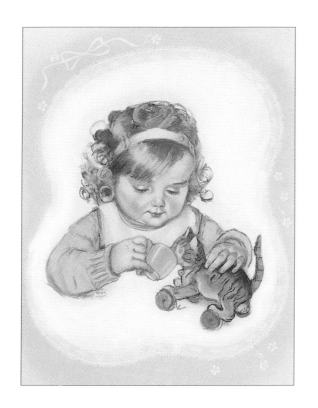

Favorite Outfit

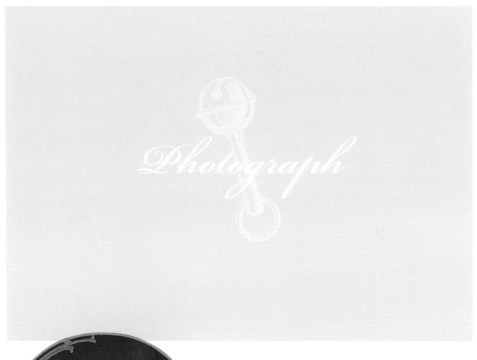

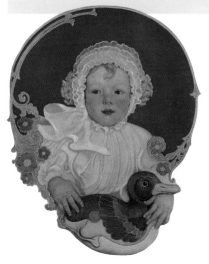

Date:

HOLIDAY MEMORIES

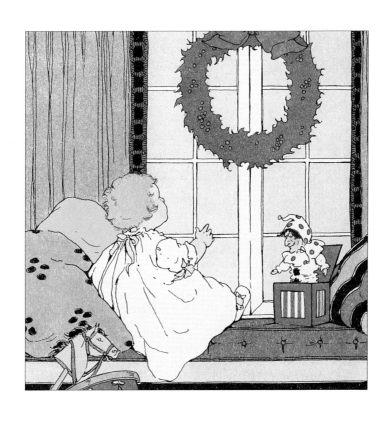

Baby's First Birthday

Date:

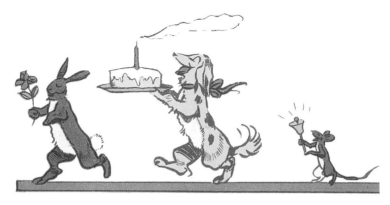

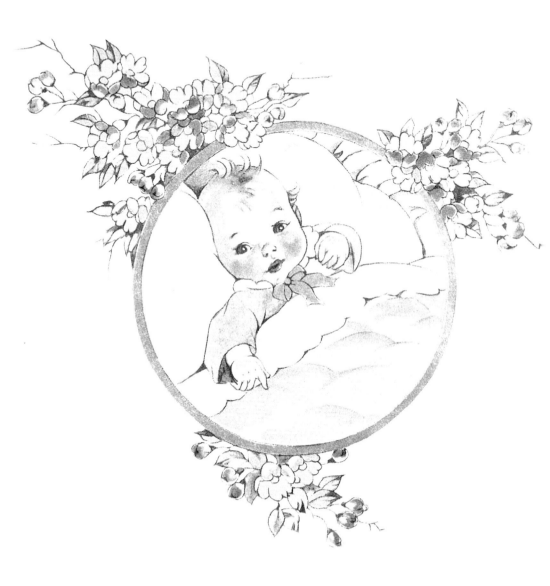

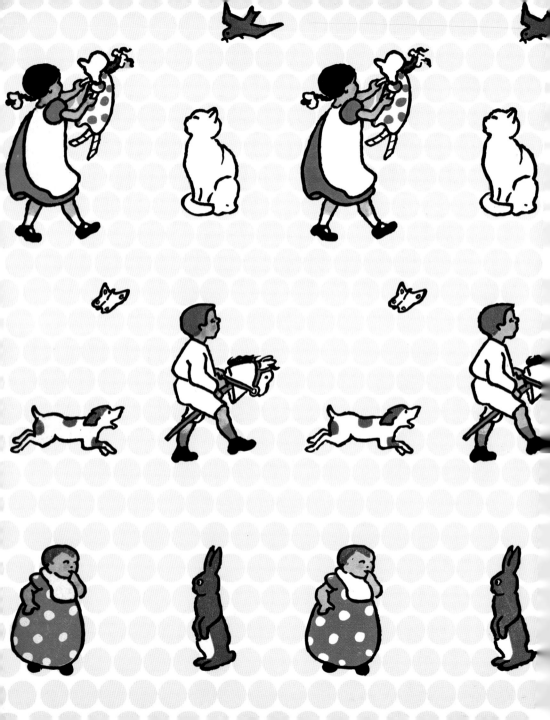